MW01298219

Contents

Pages

Preface	1-3
Conventions Used In This Book	4-5
Misery Must Be Eliminated	6-9
Vision of Yog	10-27
Breath is bigger than you	28-32
Vibrant Health and Longevity	33-44
Preparations for the Practice	45-53
The Practice	54-62
Conclusion	63-63
Index	64-65
References	66-67

Preface

Is health holding you back?
Is procrastination, laziness, doubtfulness or addiction impeding your progress?
Is misunderstanding coming in your way to success?
Is it getting hard for you to attain mastery and success?
Are setbacks preventing you from retaining success?

What do the ancient sciences of Yog and Ayurved have to offer to help with your problems?
Learn about the tools to overcome the impediments.

Preface

This book intends to inspire the readers to explore further, understand correctly and benefit from the undercurrents of the ancient sciences of India.

The intention is to connect the readers directly with the ancient seers through the unfiltered and accurate translation. And hence the book only provides translation and not the interpretation or explanation of the Sanskrit verses and Sutras.

Indian heritage is a vast ocean and this book is a small drop. Your feedback will be most welcome.
Get in touch at ravipathak@live.com or https://www.facebook.com/bharatvarsham .

Author, Ravi Pathak, is a technologist and inventor. He lives in San Francisco, USA. For 30 years he studied, practiced & benefited from Yog and Ayurved.

Conventions Used In This Book

This book uses Devanagri (देवनागरी *Devanāgarī*) to Latin transliteration from table below based on IAST standard.

Vowels	अ a	इ i	उ u	ऋ ṛ	ऌ ḷ
	आ ā	ई ī	ऊ ū	ॠ ṝ	ॡ ḹ
	ए e	ओ o	◌ं ṃ	◌ः ḥ	s `
	ऐ ai	औ au			
Consonants	क् k	ख् kh	ग् g	घ् gh	ङ् ṅ
	च् c	छ् ch	ज् j	झ् jh	ञ् ň
	ट् ṭ	ठ् ṭh	ड् ḍ	ढ् ḍh	ण् ṇ
	त् t	थ् th	द् d	ध् dh	न् n
	प् p	फ् ph	ब् b	भ् bh	म् m
	य् y	र् r	ल् l	व् v	
	श् ś	ष् ṣ	स् s	ह् h	
	क्ष् kṣ	त्र् tr	ज्ञ् jň	श्र् śr	

Conventions Used In This Book

Conventions used in this book:
1. To write Sanskrit words, three styles are used.

English (देवनागरी *Transliteration*)

Example - Om (ॐ *Oma*)

(देवनागरी *Transliteration* English)

Example - (ॐ *Oma* Om)

English (देवनागरी *Transliteration* - meaning)

Example - Om (ॐ *Oma* –Primordial sound representing God)
2. For Sanskrit verses, convention used is as follows:

Sanskrit verse in Devanagri script
Transliteration
Translation

Example:

> वसुधैव कुटुम्बकम् ॥
> ***Vasudhaiva Kuṭumbakam.***
> **Entire world is one family.**

Misery Must Be Eliminated

हेयं दुःखमनागतम् ||*2-16 Patanjali Yogasutra* ||

Heyaṁ Duḥkhamnāgatam.

The misery (दुःखम् *Duḥkham*) not yet arrived (अनागतम् *Anāgatam*) must be eliminated (हेयं *Heyaṁ*).

Misery Must Be Eliminated

व्याधिस्त्यानसंशयप्रमादालस्याविरति भ्रान्तिदर्शनं

अलब्धभूमिकत्व अनवस्थितत्वानि चित्तविक्षेपाः

ते अन्तरायाः ||*1-30 Patanjali Yogasutra* ||

Vyādhistyānasaṁśayapramādālasyāvirati Bhrāntidarśanaṁ

Alabdhabhūmikatva Anavasthitatvāni

Cittavikṣepāḥ Te Antarāyāḥ.

Disease (व्याधि *Vyādhi*), idleness (स्त्यान *Styāna*), doubtfulness (संशय *Saṁśaya*), negligence (प्रमाद *Pramāda*), lethargy (आलस्य *Ālasyā*), overindulgence (अविरति *Avirati*), misconception (भ्रान्तिदर्शनं *Bhrāntidarśanaṁ*), non-attainment of mastery (अलब्धभूमिकत्व *Alabdhabhūmikatva*) and setbacks (अनवस्थितत्व *Anavasthitatva*) are the impediments (अन्तराय *Antarāya*) (to Yoga), they are the agitators (विक्षेपाः *Vikṣepāḥ*) of the mind (चित्त *Citta*).

Misery Must Be Eliminated

दु:खदौर्मनस्याङ्गमेजयत्व श्वासप्रश्वासा विक्षेपसहभुवः

||*1-31 Patanjali Yogasutra*||

Duḥkhadaurmanasyāṅgamejayatva Śvāsapraśvāsā Vikṣepasahabhuvaḥ.

Misery (दु:ख *Duḥkha*), resentment (दौर्मनस्य *Daurmanasya*), involuntary trembling, vibrations or movements of body or limbs (अङ्गमेजयत्व *Aṅgamejayatva*), agitations of (विक्षेप *Vikṣepa*) inhalation (श्वास *Śvāsa*) and exhalation (प्रश्वास *Praśvāsā*) are born (भुवः *Bhuvaḥ*) along with (सह *Saha*) (the agitations of mind).

Misery Must Be Eliminated

तत्प्रतिषेधार्थमेकतत्त्वाभ्यासः

||*1-32 Patanjali Yogasutra*||

Tatpratiṣedhārthamekatattvābhyāsaḥ.

To remedy (प्रतिषेधार्थ *Pratiṣedhārtha*) these (तत् *Tat*), practice (अभ्यास *Abhyāsa*) one (एक *Eka*) of the precepts (तत्त्व *Tattva*) (described hereafter).

Patanjali goes on to list other precepts and then describes this one.

प्रच्छर्दनविधारणाभ्यां वा प्राणस्य ||***1-34 Patanjali Yogasutra***||

Prachardanavidhāraṇābhyāṁ Vā Prāṇasya.

Or (वा *Vā*), through the expulsion (प्रच्छर्दन *Prachardan Prachhardan*) and the accumulation (विधारण *Vidhāraṇa Vidharana*) of the breath (प्राण *Prāṇa*).

Vision Of Yog

Now follows a brief introduction of Yog.

योगश्चित्तवृत्तिनिरोधः ||***1-21 Patanjali Yogasutra***||

Yogaścittavrittinirodhaḥ.

The Yog (योग *Yoga*) is the rest (निरोध *Nirodha*) of the mind (चित्त *Citta*) from its activities (वृत्ति *Vritti*).

प्रमाण विपर्यय विकल्प निद्रा स्मृतयः ||***1-6 Patanjali Yogasutra***||

Pramāṇa Viparyaya Vikalpa Nidrā Smritayaḥ.

Verifying (प्रमाण *Pramāṇa* Proof), misunderstanding (विपर्यय *Viparyaya Reverse*), longing (विकल्प *Vikalpa* Alternative, What we don't have), sleeping (निद्रा *Nidrā Sleep*) and reminiscing (स्मृति *Smriti Memory*) (These are the five activities of mind).

Vision Of Yog

अभ्यासवैराग्याभ्यां तन्निरोधः ||***1-12 Patanjali Yogasutra***||

Abhyāsavairāgyābhyāṁ Tannirodhaḥ.

That (तत् *Tat*) (mind) is rested (निरोध *Nirodha*) through practice (अभ्यास *Abhyāsa*) and renunciation (वैराग्य *Vairāgya*).

Vision Of Yog

तत्र स्थितौ यत्नोऽभ्यासः ||*1-13 Patanjali Yogasutra*||

Tatra Sthitau Yatnobhyāsaḥ.

The effort (यत्न *Yatna*) to gain that state (स्थितौ *Sthitau*) (of rest) is called the practice (अभ्यास *Abhyāsa Abhyasa*).

Vision Of Yog

स तु दीर्घकालनैरंतर्यसत्कारसेवितो दृढ़भूमिः ||***1-14 Patanjali Yogasutra***||

Sa Tu Dīrghakālanairantaryasatkārasevito Driḍhabhūmiḥ.

That (स *Sa*) practice, only (तु *Tu*) gets firmly (दृढ़ *Driḍha*) grounded (भूमि *Bhūmi*) by lovingly (सत्कार *Satkāra*) serving (सेवित *Sevita*) it for long (दीर्घ *Dīrgha*) time (काल *Kāla*) with constancy (नैरंतर्य *Nairantarya*).

Vision Of Yog

दृष्टानुश्रविकविषयवितृष्णस्य वशीकारसंज्ञा वैराग्यम् ||*1-15 Patanjali Yogasutra*||

Driṣṭānuśravikaviṣayavitriṣṇasya Vaśīkārasaṁjñā Vairāgyam.

Having no thirst (वितृष्ण *Vitriṣṇa*) to possess (वशीकार *Vaśīkāra*) objects (विषय *Viṣaya*) the person has seen (दृष्ट *Driṣṭa*) or heard of (अनुश्रविक *Anuśravika*) is called renunciation (वैराग्य *Vairāgya Vairagya*).

Vision Of Yog

यमनियमासन प्राणायाम प्रत्याहार

धारणा ध्यान समाधयोऽष्टावङ्गानि

||*2-29 Patanjali Yogasutra*||

Yamaniyamāsana Prāṇāyāma Pratyāhāra

Dhāraṇā Dhyāna Samādhayo`ṣṭāvaṅgāni.

Yama (यम), Niyama (नियम), Asan (आसन *Āsana*), Pranayam (प्राणायाम *Prāṇāyāma*), Pratyahar (प्रत्याहार *Pratyāhāra*), Dharna (धारणा *Dhāraṇā*), Dhyan (ध्यान *Dhyāna*) and Samadhi (समाधि *Samādhi*) are the Eight Components of Yog.

Vision Of Yog

अहिंसा सत्यास्तेय ब्रह्मचर्यापरिग्रहाः यमाः ||***2-30 Patanjali Yogasutra***||

Ahiṁsā Satyāsteya Brahmacaryāparigrahāḥ Yamāḥ.

Non-violence (अहिंसा *Ahiṁsā*), truthfulness (सत्य *Satya*), non-stealing (अस्तेय *Āsteya*), continence (ब्रह्मचर्य *Brahmacarya*) and frugality (अपरिग्रह Ap*arigraha*) are the Yama.

Vision Of Yog

शौच संतोष तपः स्वाध्यायेश्वरप्रणिधानानि नियमाः ||***2-32 Patanjali Yogasutra***||

Śauca Saṁtoṣa Tapaḥ Svādhyāyeśvarpraṇidhānāni Niyamāḥ.

Cleanliness (शौच *Śauca*), contentedness (संतोष *Saṁtoṣa*), fortitude (तप *Tapa*), self study (स्वाध्याय *Svādhyāya*), dedication to God (ईश्वरप्रणिधान *Iśvarpraṇidhānān*) are the Niyama.

Vision Of Yog

स्थिरसुखमासनम् ||*2-46 Patanjali Yogasutra*||

Sthirasukhamāsanam.

Asan (आसन *Āsana*) is a posture that is steady (स्थिर *Sthira*) and pleasant (सुख *Sukha*).

प्रयत्नशैथिल्यानन्तसमापत्तिभ्याम् ||*2-47 Patanjali Yogasutra*||

Prayantnaśaithilyānantasamāpattibhyām.

Through relaxation (शैथिल्य *Śaithilya*) of the effort (प्रयत्न *Prayatna*) and meditation (समापत्ति *Samāpatti*) on the infinite (अनन्त *Ananta*) (Asan occurs).

Vision Of Yog

ततो द्वन्द्वानभिघातः ||*2-48 Patanjali Yogasutra*||

Tato Dvandvānabhighātaḥ.

(When Asan has become steady and pleasant) Then (तत *Tata*), dualities of nature (द्वन्द्व *Dvandva*) do not torment (अनभिघात *Anabhighāta*). (Dvandva represents pair of opposites like hot and cold, pleasure and sorrow, and famine and feast etc. Dvandva also means the conflict and tension with others.)

Vision Of Yog

तस्मिन् सति श्वासप्रश्वासयोर्गतिविच्छेदः प्राणायामः

||*2-49 Patanjali Yogasutra*||

Tasmin Sati Śvāsapraśvāsayorgativichedaḥ Prāṇāyāmaḥ.

(When Asan is perfected) In that state (तस्मिन् *Tasmin*), occurs (सति *Sati*) Pranayama (प्राणायाम *Prāṇāyāma*) by breaking (*Vicheda*) the natural rhythm (गति *Gati*) of inhalation (श्वास *Śvāsa*) and exhalation (प्रश्वास *Praśvāsa*).

Vision Of Yog

बाह्याभ्यन्तरस्तम्भवृत्तिः देशकालसंख्याभिः परिदृष्टो दीर्घसूक्ष्मः ||*2-50 Patanjali Yogasutra*||

Bāhyābhyantarastambhavrittiḥ
Deshkālasaṁkhyābhiḥ Paridriṣto Dīrghasukṣmaḥ.

(In the first three types of Pranayam) Outward (बाह्य *Bāhya*), inward (अभ्यन्तर *Abhyantara*) and stationary (स्तम्भ *Stambha*) states (वृत्ति *Vritti*) of the breath are regulated by the region (देश *Desh*), duration (काल *Kāla*) and count (संख्या *Saṁkhyā*), while keeping the breath deep (दीर्घ *Dīrgha*), fine (सूक्ष्म *Sukṣma*) and under observation (परिदृष्टो *Paridriṣto*).

बाह्याभ्यन्तरविषयाक्षेपी चतुर्थः ||***2-51 Patanjali Yogasutra***||

Bāhyābhyantaraviṣayākṣepī Caturthaḥ.

In the fourth (चतुर्थ *Caturtha*) Pranayam, outward (बाह्य *Bāhya*) and inward (अभ्यन्तर *Abhyantara*) breath is thrown (आक्षेपी *Ākṣepī*) at a target (विषय *Viṣaya*) i.e. breath is directed towards a target.

Vision Of Yog

ततः क्षीयते प्रकाशावरणम् ||***2-52 Patanjali Yogasutra***||

Tataḥ Kṣīyate Prakāśāvarṇam.

In that state (तत *Tata*), the veil (आवरण *Āvarṇa*) of the light (प्रकाश *Prakāśa*) is dissolved (क्षीयते *Kṣīyate*) i.e. the light of knowledge within us is unveiled.

धारणासु च योग्यता मनसः ||***2-53 Patanjali Yogasutra***||

Dharṇāsu Ca Yogyatā Manasaḥ.

And (च *Ca*), the mind (मनस *Manasa*) becomes ready for meditation (धारणा *Dharṇā Dharana*).

Vision Of Yog

स्वस्वविषयासंप्रयोगे चित्तस्य स्वरूपानुकार इवेन्द्रियाणां प्रत्याहारः ||*2-54 Patanjali Yogasutra*||

Svasvaviṣayāsaṁprayoge Cittasya Svarupānukāra Ivendriyāṇāṁ Pratyāhāraḥ.

Disengaging (असंप्रयोगे *Asaṁprayoge*) senses (इन्द्रियाणां *Indriyāṇāṁ*) from their respective (स्वस्व *Svasva*) objects (विषय *Viṣaya*) such that they start following (अनुकार *Anukāra*) the true nature (स्वरूप *Svarūpa*) of the mind (चित्त *Citta*) is Pratyahar (प्रत्याहार *Pratyāhāra*).

Vision Of Yog

देशबन्धचित्तस्य धारणा ||*3-11 Patanjali Yogasutra*||

Deśabandhacittasya Dhāraṇā.

To anchor (बन्ध *Bandha*) the mind onto one place (देश *Deśa*) is Dharna (धारणा *Dhāraṇā*).

Vision Of Yog

तत्र प्रत्ययैकतानता ध्यानम् ||*3-21 Patanjali Yogasutra*||

Tatra Pratyaikatānatā Dhyānam.

Continuous attention (एकतानता *Ekatānatā*) and knowledge (प्रत्यय *Pratyaya*) of that place (तत्र *Tatra*) is Dhyan (ध्यान *Dhyāna*).

Vision Of Yog

तदेवार्थमात्रनिर्भासं स्वरूपशून्यमिव समाधिः ||*3-31 Patanjali Yogasutra*||

Tadevārthamātranirbhāsaṁ Svarupaśūnyamiva Samādhiḥ.

Only (मात्र *Mātra*) the meaning (अर्थ *Artha*) of that place is perceived (निर्भास *Nirbhāsa*) and the perception of the own form (स्वरूप *Svarūpa*) of the seer is almost (इव *Iva*) nonexistent (शून्य *Śūnya*), then Samadhi (समाधि *Samādhi*) occurs.

This concludes the introduction of Yog. In our practice, we will be incorporating these elements of Yog.

Breath Is Bigger Than You

In the ancient Indian philosophy, all the various sciences, spirituality and religion existed in a harmonious relationship complementing each other. Surya Siddhant is an ancient treatise on the astronomy. It establishes a profound connection between human breath and rest of the universe.

षड्भिः प्राणैः विनाड़ी स्यात् तत् षष्ट्या नाड़िका स्मृता ||***Sūrya Siddhānta*** **1-11** ||

नाड़ी षष्ट्या तु नाक्षत्रमहोरात्रं प्रकीर्तितम् ||***Sūrya Siddhānta*** **1-12** ||

Ṣadbhiḥ Prāṇaiḥ Vināḍī Syāt Tat Ṣaṣṭyā Nāḍikā Smritā.

Nāḍī Ṣaṣṭyā Tu Nākṣtramahorātram.

Six Pranas become one Vinadi. Sixty Vinadis are known as one Nadi. Sixty Nadis are declared as one day on the Earth.

Breath Is Bigger Than You

One day = 24 hours = 60 Nadis

One Nadi = 24 minutes = 60 Vinadis

One Vinadi = 24 seconds = 6 Pranas

One Prana = One human breath (time during one complete inhalation and exhalation) = 4 seconds

One day = 21,600 human breaths

Thus your breath is synchronized with the movement of the planet Earth, and hence, it is synchronized with the movement of the entire universe. Entire universe is pulsating with your breath!

Breath Is Bigger Than You

Breath is the mechanism through which we exchange the cosmic life force called Prana (प्राण *Prāṇa*) with the universe. We breathe in the Prana to sustain our lives. The breath has three states – inward, outward and stationary. Inward state of the breath occurs during inhalation. Outward state of the breath occurs during exhalation. Stationary state occurs briefly when the breath reverses from inward to outward state or from outward to inward state. Stationary state is also the state of rest for the breath. Breath has two qualities – Gati (गति *Gati* Motion) and Dhriti (धृति *Dhṛti* Stability, Steadiness). The breath moves and it causes movements.

Breath Is Bigger Than You

In healthy state it is stable and steady both during the motion and during the rest. The breath is the bridge between the body and the mind. Activities happening inside the body and inside the mind, either cause disturbances or restore balance of the breath. Our goal is to maintain the stability and steadiness of the breath.

A place on the Earth's equator moves at a speed of roughly 1000 miles per hour. The Earth itself is moving around the Sun at a speed of 67,000 miles per hour. Yet, we feel that the Earth is stationary like a rock. In the same way, our breath needs to be stable and steady amidst its motion and rest.

In healthful state, the breath is deep (दीर्घ *Dīrgha* Long) and fine (सूक्ष्म *Sukṣma Sukshma* Fine, Thin, Soundless, Imperceptible). In healthful state, the breath is in a rhythmic motion (गति *Gati* Gati) and yet stable (धृति *Dhṛti* Dhriti). In healthful state, the breath is joyful (सुखी *Sukhī* Sukhi).

Breath Is Bigger Than You

To maintain good health, keep the breath under you observation (परिदृष्टो *Paridriṣto Paridrishto*) to make sure it is:

1) दीर्घ ***Dīrgha*** **Dirgha Long**
2) सूक्ष्म ***Sukṣma*** **Sukshma Fine**
3) गति ***Gati*** **Gati Rhythmic Motion**
4) धृति ***Dhṛti*** **Dhriti Stable and Steady**
5) सुखी ***Sukhī*** **Sukhi Joyful**

Vibrant Health and Longevity

Now we will consider how Ayurved views health. Ayurved (आयुर्वेद *Āyurveda*) means understanding of life (आयु *Āyu* Ayu – Life or life span, वेद *Veda* Veda – Deep understanding, true knowledge). It has been practiced in India since Vedic time going back to more than 5000 years. It originated in Rigved (ऋगवेद *Ṛgaveda*) and greatly evolved in Atharvaved (अथर्ववेद *Atharvaveda*). Then it was crystallized as treatises into two schools (1) School of Medicine and (2) School of Surgery.

Around 700 BCE, sage Charaka (चरक *Caraka*) wrote the book of medicine - Charaka Samhita (चरक संहिता *Caraka Saṁhitā*) and sage Sushrut (सुश्रुत *Suśruta*) wrote the book of surgery Sushrut Samhita (सुश्रुत संहिता *Suśruta Saṁhitā*).

Vibrant Health and Longevity

Ayurved is science of life. It provides a way of life that leads to health for long human life span of 100 years. To achieve longevity, it employs 1) Wholesome life style 2) Promotive medicine 3) Individualized medicine 4) Surgery.

Almost half of Ayurved books from Charaka and Sushrut are dedicated to wholesome lifestyle. They describe every aspect of life including diet, exercise, hygiene, adjusting diet with seasons, family life, dealing with emotions, importance of source of income and spirituality etc.

Vibrant Health and Longevity

षड्त्रिंशतं सहस्त्राणि रात्रीणां हितभोजनः।
जीवत्यनातुरो जन्तुर्जितात्मा सम्मतः सताम् ॥
1.27.348 *Caraka Saṁhita* ॥

Ṣadtriṁśataṁ Sahastrāṇi Rātrīṇāṁ Hitbhojanaḥ,
Jīvatyanāturo Janturjitātmā Sammataḥ Satām.

One who feeds on wholesome diet and conducts life with restraints approved by wise; lives peacefully for 100 years.

Italian explorer Marco Polo of Venice visited India in the year 1292 CE. He was awed by the longevity of the Indian people he met and he wrote in his book The Travels of Marco Polo - "They are extremely long-lived, every man of them living to 150 or 200 years. They eat very little, but what they do eat is good".

Vibrant Health and Longevity

Ayurved emphasizes the importance of moderate exercise combined with rest and relaxation.

व्यायामस्विन्नगात्रस्य पद्भ्यामुद्वितितस्य च।
व्याधयो नोपसर्पन्ति सिंहं क्षुद्रमृगा इव ॥ **4.24.43**

Suśruta Saṁhita ॥

Vyāyāmsvinnagātrasya Padbhyāmudvirtitasya C,
Vyādhayo Nopasarpanti Siṁhaṁ Kṣudramṛgā Iva.

Diseases do not approach the person who sweats his body with exercise and relaxes the body with massage; as small animals like deer do not come near the lion.

Vibrant Health and Longevity

शरीरायासजननं कर्म व्यायामसञ्ज्ञितम्।

तत् कृत्वा तु सुखं देहं विमृद्नीयात् समन्ततः ॥

4.24.38 *Suśruta Saṁhita* ॥

Śarīrāyāsajananaṁ Karma Vyāyāmasaňjňitam, Tat Kṛtvā Tu Sukhaṁ Dehaṁ Vimṛdnīyāt Samantataḥ.

Action generated by the physical effort of the body is called Vyayama (व्यायाम *Vyāyāma* Exercise). Massage the entire body (after the exercise). By doing that, the body becomes happy.

Vibrant Health and Longevity

बलस्यार्धेन कर्तव्यो व्यायामो हन्त्यतोऽन्यथा ।
हृदि स्थानस्थितो वायुर्यदा वक्त्रं प्रपद्यते ॥

***Suśruta Saṁhita* 4.24.47 ॥**

Balasyārdhena Kartavyo Vyāyāmo Hantyato`nyathā,
Hṛdi Sthānasthito Vāyuryadā Vaktraṁ Prapadyate.

Exercise only up to half of your power; more is injurious. Stop exercising when the breath naturally residing in the chest begins to flow from the mouth.

Vibrant Health and Longevity

To expedite the journey to attain the perfect health, we will employ four components:

1) Physical Activity

2) Rest

3) Light Meal

4) Happiness

1) Physical Activity: Integrate moderate physical activity in your daily life. Any physical activity that you enjoy will do like walking, swimming, hiking, biking or sports etc. The activity you choose must result into light sweating and must leave you energized and refreshed. There is substantial evidence based on medical research that walking 10,000 steps daily has measurable health benefits. It can be the sum total of the steps you take during the day.

2) Rest: Always be in the state of restfulness. Take breaks from the work to rest. Try few minutes of nap during the day. Sleep adequately. Start with 8 hours of sleep every night. Experiment with longer or shorter sleeping hours to find out the optimal number of hours of sleep that leaves you composed and energized next day.

3) Light Meal: Take light meals. Start by reducing your meal portions. Figure out the meal portion that provides you with adequate energy without over filling you.

त्रिविधं कुक्षौ स्थापयेदवकाशांशमाहारस्याहारमुपयुञ्जानः; तद्यथा- एकमवकाशांशं मूर्तानामाहारविकाराणाम्, एकं द्रवाणाम्, एकं पुनर्वातपित्तश्लेष्मणाम्; एतावतीं ह्याहारमात्रामुपयुञ्जानो नामात्राहारजं किञ्चिदशुभं प्राप्नोति ||**3.2.3** ***Caraka Saṁhita*** ||

Trividhaṁ Kukṣau Sthāpayedavakaśāṁśamāhāramupayuňjānaḥ;

Tadyathā - Ekamavakāśāṁśaṁ Mūrtānāmāhāravikārāṇām, Ekaṁ Dravāṇām, Ekaṁ Punarvātapittaśleṣmaṇām; Ekāvatīṁ Hyāhāramātrāmūpayuňjāno Nāmātrāhāraja Kiňcidśubhaṁ Prāpnoti.

Vibrant Health and Longevity

To consume the meal, allocate the space in the belly into three portions – in such a way that – one portion is allocated for solid food, one portion is allocated for liquids and one portion is allocated for Vata, Pitta and Kapha (or digestive process). Taking meal in such quantity, consumer is not inflicted with the harmful effects caused by the food taken in inappropriate quantity.

4) Happiness:

समदोषः समाग्निश्च समधातुमलक्रियः ।

प्रसन्नात्मेन्द्रियमनाः स्वस्थ इत्यभिधीयते ||**1.15.41**

Suśruta Saṁhita ||

Samdoṣaḥ Smāgniśca Samdhātumalakriyaḥ,

Prasannātmendriyamanāḥ Swastha Ityabhidhīyate.

When the body Doshas (Vata, Pitta and Kapha) are in equilibrium, body heat is in equilibrium and body tissues are in equilibrium, and body regularly produces waste products, and the self, the senses and the mind are in the state of happiness, then the person is declared healthy.

According to Ayurved, happiness is necessary for the person to become healthy.

Vibrant Health and Longevity

One of the most revered books in India, Bhagwat Gita, says:

प्रसादे सर्वदुःखानां हानिरस्योपजायते,

प्रसन्नचेतसो ह्याशु बुद्धिः पर्यवतिष्ठते ||**2.65 *Bhāgvat Gita***||

Prasāde Sarvaduḥkhānāṁ Hānirasyopajāyate,

Prasannacetaso Hyaśu Buddhiḥ Paryavatiṣṭhate.

Through the happiness, all sorrows are destroyed. Definitely, happy person's intellect is quickly established.

In order to gain perfect health, practice to be happy. Constantly remind yourself to be happy. Practice it with effort till happiness becomes your habit.

Preparations For The Practice

1) **Asan:** Asan (आसन *Āsana*) means both the seat and the seating posture. Always do Pranayam while sitting. Ideally sit on a Yoga mat or on a woolen shawl or sheet spread on the floor. Seat should be firm, level and comfortable.

Pranayam is best done while sitting in an Asan. Sukhasan is adequate. If it is physically not possible to sit in an Asan, then you can sit on a chair and keep the feet on the woolen shawl or sheet spread on the ground. For Sukhasan, sit in a cross-legged posture and stretch both arms over the knees, palms facing upwards. Arms and your body make a nice pyramid. Back should be straight. Back, neck and head should be aligned along a vertical line.

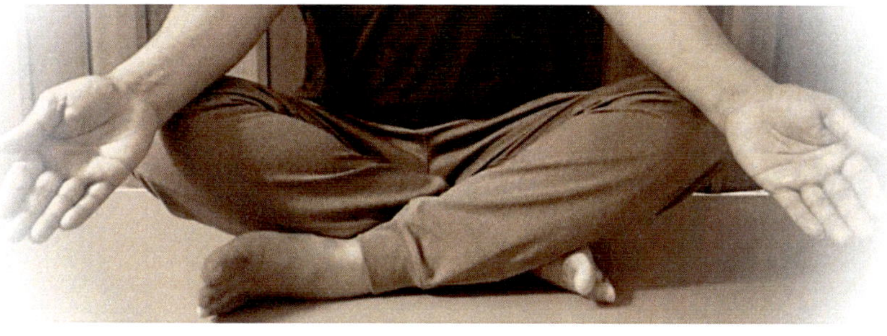

Preparations For The Practice

Those who want to get rid of the muscular aches and pains can fold their index finger burying the index finger in the root of the thumb and pressing it gently by the thumb while keeping the remaining three fingers open and straight.

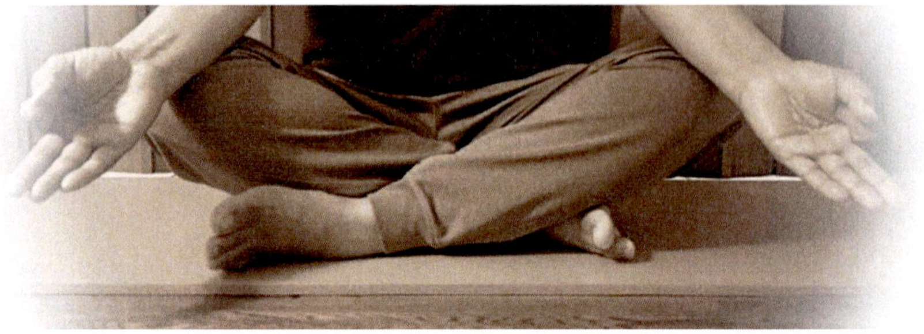

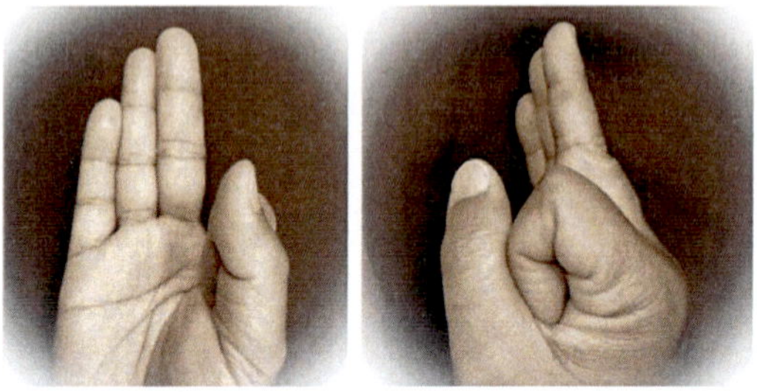

In Asan, body needs to be still and steady. Stillness and steadiness will come from daily practice. When there is a physical urge that needs body movement, do what is needed and then resume the practice. With constant daily practice such urges will go away.

Preparations For The Practice

2) Place: Select a place that is clean, quiet and away from distractions. Place should provide comfortable ambient temperature and ventilation. Open the window to get fresh air.

3) Time: Empty stomach before breakfast is ideal for Pranayam. For the best outcome brush your teeth, have a bowel movement, take a shower and before eating breakfast practice the Pranayam. After the Pranayam wait for at least 15 minutes before having a meal. Pranayam should be completed at least three hours before going to bed.

Preparations For The Practice

4) **Duration:** Practice the Pranayam for 6 minutes in one sitting. In the beginning, it may be uncomfortable to sit for 6 minutes. When you get tired then take a brief break for couple of minutes and then resume. Increase the time by 6 minutes every week or with the pace you feel comfortable. Later on, as you get comfortable, then you can practice one sitting in the morning for 30 minutes and one sitting in the evening for 30 minutes.

5) **Continuity:** Yogic skills are perfected over long time with daily practice. Continue with the Pranayam for at least three months to gain the full benefits. If you miss the practice, resume it at the next daily practice time. If during or after the practice, you notice a discomfort that does not go away or gets worse, then pause the practice for few days. It is an indication that you are not practicing in the right way or you are putting too much effort. Observe, evaluate and resume the practice when you feel comfortable.

Preparations For The Practice

6) **Precautions:** If you are a female and may be pregnant, then do not practice this Pranayam. If you have any stomach related disorder or any disorder in the organs of abdominal, pelvic or chest region do not practice this Pranayam. Always consult your primary care physician or family doctor or the doctor who provides you medical care before starting and during this practice. This Pranayam is not designed to treat medical conditions.

7) **Rest:** Pranayam should be followed by a relaxation exercise. Lie down on the Yoga mat with back flat on the mat. Keep your feet one foot apart. Keep hands on the mat and slightly away from the body, palms facing upwards. Jiggle your body gently to settle it in comfortable position. Close your eyes. Bring your awareness to the right leg. Keeping your attention to the right leg, mentally say –"I relax my right leg. My entire right leg is relaxed. My right leg is completely relaxed, healthy and happy. Thank you my right leg, I love you". Repeat the same process for each part of your

body one by one. After the right leg, bring your attention to the left leg. Repeat the process for the left leg. Then bring your attention to the organs of excretion and reproduction. Repeat the process. Then move to the abdomen, stomach and chest. Then move to the waist, lower back and upper back. Then move to the right hand and shoulder. Then move to the left hand and shoulder. Repeat the process for each part so far. Then move to the face. Mentally say –"I relax my chin, I relax my upper lip, lower lip, teeth and tongue. I relax my right cheek and jaw. I relax my right ear. I relax my left cheek and jaw. I relax my left ear. I relax my left nostril. I relax my right nostril. I relax my nose. I relax my right eye brow. I relax my right eye. I relax my right eye brow. I relax my right eye. I relax my right forehead. I relax my left forehead. I relax my head. I relax my hair. I relax my entire face. My entire face is relaxed. My face is completely relaxed, healthy and happy. I love you my face, thank you". Then bring your awareness to the entire body. Mentally say - "I relax my body. My entire body is relaxed. My body is completely relaxed, healthy and happy. Thank you my body, I love you”. Be in this relaxed state for few moments. Then turn on your right side. Slowly rise and sit cross legged. Rub your palms for few seconds. Cover your eyes with palms for about a minute till the warmth of palms fade away. Now slowly open your eyes. Relaxation exercise is completed.

8) **Be Gentle:** Yogic methods are perfected when the last remaining effort is eliminated. Make your practice effortless, natural and easy. During the Pranayam the breath should flow smoothly, steadily, naturally and effortlessly. When an effort is required, make it gentle. Outcome of the Pranayam depends on the duration of the practice, the extent of your attention on the practice and the continuity on daily basis. Effort can slow down the progress. Let go of the effort. When the effort is needed, make it gentle. Expelling air too hard or too forcefully during Prachhardan can cause fatigue, headache or injury.

Preparations For The Practice

9) Pranayam Cycle:

प्रच्छर्दनविधारणाभ्यां वा प्राणस्य ||*1-34 Patanjali Yogasutra*||

Prachardanavidhāraṇābhyāṁ Vā Prāṇasya.

Or (वा *Vā*), through the expulsion (प्रच्छर्दन *Prachardan*) and the accumulation (विधारण *Vidhāraṇa*) of the breath (प्राण *Prāṇa*).

Breath alternates between two actions in this Pranayam. First action is Prachhardan when we expel the air rapidly and profusely. During this action, lower abdominal muscles between navel and four finger widths below the navel contract. Air is rapidly and profusely thrown out through nostrils. Rushing out air makes a perceptible gentle sound. Effort is brief, gentle and comfortable.

After the Prachhardan, breath becomes ready for transition to inwards movement. There is a brief period, ever so short, for this transition.

Preparations For The Practice

Let it occur naturally. Then second action starts and the breath starts gently flowing inwards. Incoming breath is slow, steady and quiet. As breath accumulates, abdominal muscles slowly and gently expand. This accumulation action is called Vidharana. Vidharana is completed when air is comfortably filled in the lungs and belly is naturally expanded to a comfortable and natural state. At this point in time, the breath becomes ready for transition to Prachhardan. There is a brief period, ever so short, for this transition. Let it occur naturally. Then do the Prachhardan. Thus the cycle of Prachhardan and Vidharana continues. The breath continues through this cycle of Prachhardan and Vidharana with ever so gentle transition delineating them.

The Practice

Spread your Asan (seat) – Yoga mat or a woolen sheet on the floor. Open the window, if you are indoors. Sit comfortably in Sukhasan on the Asan facing the window. (You can sit on the chair with feet firmly on the ground above a woolen sheet.). Sit up tall with back straight, eyes gazing straight in the front, and back and head aligned in a straight line. Set the timer on your phone or a timer device for the Pranayam.

The Practice

Close your eyes. Bring your awareness to the right leg. Keeping your attention to the right leg, mentally say –"I relax my right leg. My right leg is completely relaxed". Repeat the same process for each part of your body one by one. After the right leg, bring your attention to the left leg. Repeat the process for the left leg. Then bring your attention to the organs of excretion and reproduction. Repeat the process. Then move to the abdomen, stomach and chest. Then move to the waist, lower back and upper back. Then move to the right hand and shoulder. Then move to the left hand and shoulder. Repeat the process for each part so far. Then move to the face. Mentally say –"I relax my chin, I relax my upper lip, lower lip, teeth and tongue. I relax my right cheek and jaw. I relax my right ear. I relax my left cheek and jaw. I relax my left ear. I relax my left nostril. I relax my right nostril. I relax my nose. I relax my right eye brow. I relax my right eye. I relax my left eye brow. I relax my left eye. I relax my right forehead. I relax my left forehead. I relax my head. I relax my hair. I relax my entire face. My face is completely relaxed". Then bring your awareness to the entire body. Mentally say - "I relax my body. My entire body is relaxed. My body is completely relaxed".

Mentally say –"I am connected with the entire universe, the infinite universe. I am united with the infinite universe. Wherever I see, I see infinite and only infinite. I am merged with this infinite. I am infinite".

Remind yourself to sit up tall with back straight, and back and head aligned in a straight line.

Keep your eyes closed during the practice.

The Practice

Take a deep breath. Breathe out with Prachhardan. Observe the lower abdominal muscles between navel and four finger widths below the navel contract. Observe the air that is rapidly and profusely thrown out through the nostrils. Observe the brief period, ever so short, for the transition as the breath turns to flow inwards. Let it occur naturally. Then breathe in with Vidharana. Incoming breath is slow, steady and quiet. As the breath accumulates, abdominal muscles slowly and gently expand. Observe that air is comfortably filled in the lungs and belly is naturally expanded to a comfortable and natural state. The breath now becomes ready for transition to Prachhardan. There is a brief period, ever so short, for this transition. Let it occur naturally. Then do the Prachhardan. Repeat this cycle for few times.

The Practice

During next Prachhardan, mentally say "Prachhardan". During Vidharana, mentally say "Vidharana". Repeat this for few times.

After next Prachhardan, mentally say *"Paridrishto"* and observe the breathing till the next Prachhardan. Repeat this cycle for few times.

After next Prachhardan, mentally say "Dirgha" and observe the breathing till the next Prachhardan. Observe that breathing is deep. Repeat this cycle for few times.

After next Prachhardan, mentally say "Sukshma" and observe the breathing till the next Prachhardan. Observe that breathing is slow, quiet, steady and fine. Repeat this cycle for few times.

After next Prachhardan, mentally say *"Paridrishto* Dirgha Sukshma" and observe the breathing till the next Prachhardan. Observe that breathing is deep and fine. Repeat this cycle for few times.

The Practice

After next Prachhardan, mentally say *"Vidharana"* and observe the breathing till the next Prachhardan. Observe that the air is comfortably filled in the lungs and belly is naturally expanded to a comfortable and natural state. Now the breath becomes ready for transition to Prachhardan. There is a brief period, ever so short, for this transition. Let it occur naturally. Then do the Prachhardan. Repeat this cycle for few times.

Remind yourself to sit up tall with back straight, and back and head aligned in a straight line.

After next Prachhardan, mentally say "Pranayami Sukhi Bhaveta" (प्राणायामी सुखी भवेत *Prāṇāyāmī Sukhī Bhaveta* The one who is doing Pranayam is becoming joyful) or mentally say "I am feeling happy". Feel that you are filling with joy as Vidharana naturally progresses. After Vidharana, do the Prachhardan. Repeat this cycle for the remainder of the practice time. (If you are using a timer, set it at the low volume).

The Practice

Now switch your hands to the relaxing pose, palms comfortably resting on the knees.

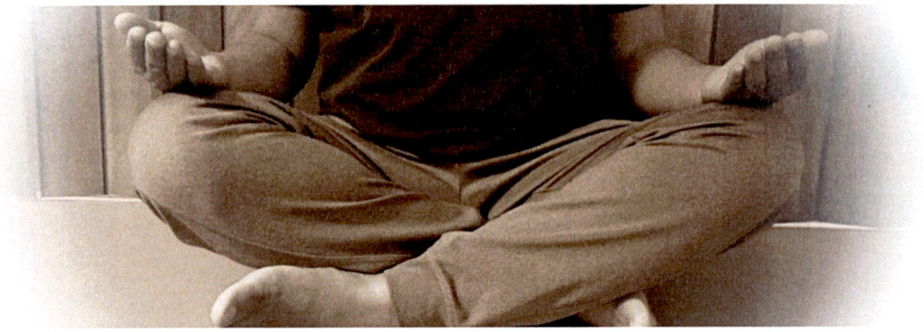

Sit with eyes closed for some time. Observe the breath as it occurs naturally. Breathing is happening by itself. You are only observing the breath. Breathing is happening naturally, you are only observing it. Keep observing the breath as long as you feel like.

The Practice

Keep your eyes closed. Now you are ready to do the relaxation exercise. Lie down on the Yoga mat with back flat on the mat. Keep your feet one foot apart. Keep hands on the mat and slightly away from the body, palms facing upwards. Jiggle your body gently to settle it in comfortable position. Close your eyes. Bring your awareness to the right leg. Keeping your attention to the right leg, mentally say –"I relax my right leg. My entire right leg is relaxed. My right leg is completely relaxed, healthy and happy. Thank you my right leg, I love you". Repeat the same process for each part of your body one by one. After the right leg, bring your attention to the left leg. Repeat the process for the left leg. Then bring your attention to the organs of excretion and reproduction. Repeat the process. Then move to the abdomen, stomach and chest. Then move to the waist, lower back and upper back. Then move to the right hand and shoulder. Then move to the left hand and shoulder. Repeat the process for each part so far. Then move to the face. Mentally say –"I relax my chin, I relax my upper lip, lower lip, teeth and tongue. I relax my right cheek and jaw. I relax my right ear. I relax my left cheek and jaw. I relax my left ear. I relax my left nostril. I relax my right nostril. I relax my nose. I relax my right eye brow. I relax my right eye. I relax my right eye brow. I relax my right eye. I relax my right forehead. I relax my left forehead. I relax my head. I relax my hair. I relax my entire face. My entire face is relaxed. My face is completely relaxed, healthy and happy. I love you my face, thank you". Then bring your awareness to the entire body. Mentally say - "I relax my body. My entire body is relaxed. My body is completely relaxed, healthy and happy. Thank you my body, I love you". Be in this relaxed state for few moments. Then turn on your right side. Slowly rise and sit cross legged. Rub your palms for few seconds. Cover your eyes with palms for about a minute till the warmth of palms fade away. Now slowly open your eyes. Relaxation exercise is completed. This also completes your practice session.

Conclusion

Yogic practices take time to yield results. Stick with this practice for at least three months. Slowly increase the duration from 6 minutes in the increments of 6 minutes per week or longer. Be comfortable with the pace. Be gentle in the effort. With any exercise, there is some soreness or discomfort in the beginning that goes away. If you experience discomfort, pause the practice. Take a break and evaluate the pace and the effort. Make it gentler and proceed. Take a break for a few minutes & up to a couple of days. Consult your doctor before starting the practice and during the three months of initial practice as needed. Incorporate some physical activity in daily routine, get adequate sleep and continue the daily practice. Sanskrit word for healthy is Svastha (स्वस्थ *Svastha).* स्व Sva means self, थ Tha means to settle or to dwell. A person settled in the self is healthy. When this ease is disturbed disease follows. When this order is disturbed disorder follows. This practice unites and settles the person with the self. It makes the person centered. It restores ease and order between the person and the person’s innate nature.

Index

A

Abhyasa · 12
Aryabhata Siddhanta · 66
Asan · 18
Atharvaved · 33
Ayurved · 33

B

Be Gentle · 51

C

Charak · 33

D

Devanagri · 4
Dharana · 23
Dhriti · 32
Dhyan · 26
Dirgha · 32

E

Eight Components of Yog · 15

G

Gati · 32

M

Marco Polo · 35
Mimansasutra · 67

N

Niyama · 17
Nyaysutra · 66

P

Patanjali · 6, 7
Prachardana · 9
Prana · 30
Pranayam Cycle · 52
Pranayama · 20
Pranayami Sukhi Bhaveta · 59
Pratyahar · 24

R

Rest · 49
Rigved · 33

Index

S

Samadhi · 27
Sankhyasutra · 66
Sukhi · 32
Sukshma · 32
Sushrut · 33
Svastha · 63

T

The Travels of Marco Polo · 35

V

Vairagya · 14
Vaisheshiksutra · 66
Vidharana · 9

Y

Yama · 16
Yog · 10
Yogasutra · 67

References

A. Aryabhatiyam (आर्यभटीयम् *Āryabhaṭīyam*)

B. Aryabhata Siddhanta (आर्यभट सिद्धांत *Āryabhaṭa Siddhānta*)

C. Surya Siddhanta (सूर्य सिद्धान्त *Sūrya Siddhānta*)

D. Shrimadbhagwat Gita (श्रीमद्भागवत् गीता *Sṛīmadabhāgavat Gītā*)

E. Shrimadbhagwat Mahapuran (श्रीमद्भागवत् महापुराण *Sṛīmadabhāgavat Mahāpurāṇa*)

F. Vishnu Puran (विष्णु पुराण *Viṣṇu Purāṇa*)

G. Charaka Samhita (चरक संहिता *Carak Saṁhitā)*

H. Sushrut Samhita (सुश्रुत संहिता *Suśruta Saṁhitā*)

I. Gheranda Samhita (घेरण्ड संहिता *Gheraṇḍa Saṁhitā*)

J. Hathayog Pradipika (हठयोग प्रदीपिका *Haṭhayoga Pradīpikā*)

K. Nyaysutra (न्यायसूत्र *Nyāyasūtra*)

L. Sankhyasutra (सांख्यसूत्र *Sāṁkhyasūtra*)

M. Vaisheshiksutra (वैशेषिकसूत्र *Vaiśeṣikasūtra*)

References

N. Mimansasutra (मीमांसासूत्र *Mīmāṁsāsūtra*)

O. Yogasutra (योगसूत्र *Yogasūtra*)

P. Goraksha Paddhati (गोरक्ष पद्धति *Gorakṣa Paddhati*)

Disclaimer: A healthcare professional should be consulted to treat your specific medical situations. The authors and the publishers disclaim any and all liability arising directly or indirectly from the use or application of any information contained in this book. Information provided in the book is for the informational purposes only and any use of the information contained in this book is at the discretion of the reader.

21734849R00038

Made in the USA
San Bernardino, CA
04 January 2019